UNDERSTANDING EHLERS-DANLOS SYNDROME

GENETICS, DIAGNOSIS AND LIVING WITH EHLERS-DANLOS SYNDROME

Nikole J. Daly

Table Of Content

Introduction To Ehlers-Danlos Syndrome	1
Types of Ehlers-Danlos Syndrome	9
Signs and Symptoms of Ehlers-Danlos Syndrome	16
Affected Populace	24
Correlated conditions	34
Associated disorder	45
Root Causes	50
Preventive Strategies	59
Diagnosis Process	70
Therapeutic Approaches (treatment)	83
Alternative treatment Approaches	97
Ideal Diet for Managing Ehlers-Danlos Syndrome	111
Foods to Steer Clear of	133
Physical Activities (Exercises)	156
Guidance for Coping with the Condition	172
Conclusion	187

Copyright © 2023 **Nikole J. Daly**

All Rights Reserved.

Before this copy is duplicated or reproduced in any manner, the publisher's consent must be gained. Therefore, the contents within can neither be stored electronically, transferred, nor kept in a database. Neither in part nor full can the document be copied, scanned, faxed or retained without approval from the publisher or creator

CHAPTER 1

INTRODUCTION TO EHLERS-DANLOS SYNDROME (EDS)

The Ehlers-Danlos syndrome is a kind of hypermobility disorder that is passed down through families very seldom and damages the body's connective tissues. These tissues are akin to the scaffolding that provides structure and support to many parts of the body, including as the skin, joints, blood vessels, and even organs. Some of these parts include the articulations of the joints and the blood arteries.

Collagen, a protein that works as a structural component for these connective tissues, is an essential component of this process as well as an essential actor. Collagen acts as a structural component.

Collagen functions in a manner similar to that of the foundation and walls of a building in that it binds all of the other components together. Because to Ehlers-Danlos syndrome, these LEGO bricks do not always fit together in the proper manner, which leads to connections that are weaker.

There are multiple different subtypes of Ehlers-Danlos syndrome, and each of these subtypes is distinguished by a different grouping of symptoms. One of the characteristics that are shared by many different types is called hypermobility, and it refers to joints that have the ability to move farther than the normal range of motion for particular joints. For instance, you could bend your fingers so that they point in the other way, or your knees could extend farther than they normally would.

In spite of the fact that this could give the impression of being a superhero, it really raises the likelihood of feeling pain, joint dislocations, and finally arthritis.

Another essential component of the body is the epidermis. People who have Ehlers-Danlos syndrome may have skin that is notably smoother and more velvety than the ordinary person's skin. It is capable of stretching more than typical skin, which may sound exciting, but if it is not properly cared for, it may lead to issues.

Because they have an influence on the cardiovascular system, including the blood vessels and the heart, some kinds of Ehlers-Danlos syndrome are especially harmful. This is because the cardiovascular system is responsible for blood circulation throughout the body. Consider the blood veins in your body to be like highways, delivering blood to all the different sections of your body.

Some forms of Ehlers-Danlos Syndrome may cause these "highways" to become weaker, which can lead to potential risks such as aneurysms, which are bulges in blood arteries, or even the possibility of organ rupture.

Because Ehlers-Danlos syndrome may be inherited, the first thing a doctor would often do is investigate the patient's family history. This is because EDS may be inherited. It is impossible to overestimate the significance of physical examinations; during these examinations, medical professionals check for signs such as hypermobility and elastic skin. Genetic testing may also be used to identify the specific forms of Ehlers-Danlos syndrome that an individual has.

In order to properly manage Ehlers-Danlos syndrome, one has to implement a plan that consists of many components. In this setting, the use of physical therapy is very necessary. It is the same as having a personal trainer give you workouts to strengthen your muscle endurance and provide extra support for your arthritic joints. In other words, it is the comparable. This might make the pain you're feeling a little bit better, and it could also generally boost your mobility.

The use of splints or braces that have been fabricated on an individual basis may be recommended in certain instances. By using these external supports, damage to joints that are already unstable may be prevented, and the joints themselves can be stabilized.

When living with Ehlers-Danlos syndrome, it is essential to exercise a certain level of caution at all times. It's probable that individuals who have Ehlers-Danlos syndrome may need to make certain changes to the way they go about their day-to-day lives in order to accommodate the disease. Imagine playing your favorite sport if you had Ehlers-Danlos

Syndrome; you may need to modify the rules of the game in order to avoid undue stress from being placed on your joints.

It is crucial to have the awareness that a person's worth or skills are not dependant on having the disease even if there is presently no therapy available for Ehlers-Danlos Syndrome (EDS). People who have Ehlers-Danlos syndrome are able to have fulfilling lives if they get the required medical care, take part in the appropriate physical therapy, and make the necessary adjustments to their way of living.

They learn the abilities required to overcome the special challenges they experience and come to grips with the distinctive pattern of their bodies. This allows them to advance in their quest.

CHAPTER 2

TYPES OF EHLERS-DANLOS SYNDROME (EDS)

The Ehlers-Danlos syndrome is analogous to a complex jigsaw puzzle due to the fact that it is made up of many diverse pieces. Because every component is its own special form of EDS, the completed body will never be precisely the same, even if it is made from the same materials.

1. Extremely mobile Ehlers-Danlos Syndrome, also known as hEDS People who have this form of EDS are able to do acts that others are unable to, such as bending their fingers or

arms in strange directions. Others who do not have this form of EDS are unable to perform these actions. On the other hand, due to the great pliability of their joints, they have to exercise tremendous care in order to protect themselves from sustaining injuries. It's possible that the joints in their body can even dislocate at times, which can be a very painful experience.

2. The conventional EDS, often known as the cEDS: Imagine that your skin is fabric that you can manipulate. Patients who have cEDS have compromised skin because the "fabric" of their skin has been damaged, which makes their skin less robust than it should be. It may

be easily torn or bruised, just as paper can. Similar to paper. It is possible for people who have cEDS to have skin that is velvety or has a texture that is similar to velvet. It is possible that their joints have some degree of pliability, but not even close to as much as those of hEDS. They might sometimes have troubles with their eyes or their spine.

3. Vascular EDS vEDS: This form affects the organs as well as the blood vessels. People who are living with vEDS need to take an excessive amount of care since the illness may cause problems with their blood vessels. They might be at a larger risk for some things, such

as a tear in one of their blood vessels, which could lead to serious issues with their health.

4. Kyphoscoliotic EDS (kEDS): This kind of EDS may have an impact on the maturation of your spine (the bones in your back) as you become older. Other people who have KEDS may have a curved spine, which may lead them to walk in a way that is distinct from the method in which people who do not have the disease walk. In addition to this, it's possible that their muscles aren't as powerful as they once were, and that they have trouble with their eyes.

5. Arthrochalasia EDS (aEDS): If you have aEDS, it is possible that your joints will not stay in place the way they should. It's likely that children born to mothers who have been exposed to AEDs will have hips that don't quite have the right form. Individuals who have had this sort of damage may be more prone to damaging their joints and dislocating them in the future.

6. Dermatosparaxis EDS (dEDS): People who have dEDS may have skin that is very sensitive and loose, which makes it more prone to ripping readily. In addition to this, their skin may have an increased quantity of wrinkles. Because their skin is not as thick or

tough as the skin of other individuals, it may take longer for wounds to heal on them than it does on other people.

7. More of a variety: There are a few more, less frequent forms of Ehlers-Danlos syndrome in addition to these basic subtypes of the disorder that are often seen. Because of the distinct characteristics that each individual has, individuals may be distinguished from one another. Some strains, for example, are known to interfere with the typical operation of a person's muscles, while others are known to have an effect on a person's ability to hear.

Keep in mind that persons who have Ehlers-Danlos Syndrome are one of a kind, and despite the fact that their bodies may seem slightly different, they are still remarkable despite these differences. Despite the fact that their bodies may appear somewhat different, they are one of a kind.

CHAPTER 3

SIGNS AND SYMPTOMS OF EHLERS-DANLOS SYNDROME (EDS)

1. Extremely Stretchy Skin People who have Ehlers-Danlos Syndrome have the capacity to perform a movement like this with their skin. This is one of the defining characteristics of the condition. They may be able to pull it for a decent distance, but it has the elastic quality of returning to its starting location after being moved. As a consequence of this, the appearance of their skin may be noticeably dissimilar from that of other individuals. There are also tales that their skin may

sometimes have a texture that is quite similar to velvet.

2. Flexible Joints: Individuals who have Ehlers-Danlos Syndrome often have joints that are more movable than they should be. This is a symptom of the syndrome. It's possible that their limbs may bend in ways that catch you by complete surprise. Because of this, it is possible that they may become highly good in sports such as gymnastics; nevertheless, it is also possible that it could cause their joints to suffer on occasion.

3. Blemishes That Are Easily Distributed Spots of these hues are more likely to form on the

skin of people who have Ehlers-Danlos syndrome than those without the condition. They are prone to obtaining scratches and bruises from things that most people would not ordinarily be injured by, such as materials that are generally innocuous. Their skin is quite delicate, and it creases and wrinkles easily due to its thinness and fragility.

4. A Sluggish Recovery The healing process for a wound, such as a cut or scrape, starts practically immediately after the injury occur in the body. Those who suffer from Ehlers-Danlos Syndrome, on the other hand, may have a slower recovery time after being injured. It is almost as if their bodies need a

little bit of more time in order to properly place everything where it should be.

5. Suffering from pain in the joints Joint pain is a common symptom of Ehlers-Danlos syndrome, which may be experienced by affected individuals. It's a little like having an upset stomach, except the discomfort is concentrated in their joints rather than in their stomachs.

6. The Sensation That the Skin Is Fragile People who have Ehlers-Danlos Syndrome may have the experience of their skin feeling as if it is fragile. It just takes a little impact from another item for it to become readily torn

apart. There is a possibility that their skin has a texture that is unusually smooth and silky.

7. People who have Ehlers-Danlos syndrome could have feet that are flatter than typical, which might give the impression that the feet are collapsing more than usual while the person is standing. As a consequence of this element, they may sometimes have the sensation that walking is not the same for them.

8. Difficulties Associated with the Muscles It's possible that people who have Ehlers-Danlos syndrome have muscles that feel like they're wasting away more quickly or that have a

weakening feeling. It is the same as having muscles that do not want to work as hard as they typically would. Having this condition is the same thing.

9. Difficulties relating to the eyes People who have Ehlers-Danlos syndrome often have eyes that are more sensitive to the feeling of light. This symptom may occur at any moment. It's feasible that they may see more clearly if they used glasses instead of their current contact lenses. In addition, their eyes may have the sensation of being dry or uncomfortable.

10. A curved spine People who have Ehlers-Danlos syndrome may sometimes have a

curved spine. They nearly give off the impression of having a curved back rather than a straight back.

11. Difficulties Associated with the Digestive System People who have Ehlers-Danlos syndrome may have problems with their digestive system, more specifically with their stomach or intestines. It's probable that they get stomach pains more often than other people.

12. Concerns Relating to the Heart In certain people, the Ehlers-Danlos syndrome may lead to heart-related complications. It is possible that the heart will perform abnormally as a

result of this compared to how it normally would. If one want to keep their heart in good health, it is imperative that they seek the advice of trained medical specialists.

Keep in mind that no two puzzles are the same, and despite the fact that persons with Ehlers-Danlos syndrome may have pieces that are different from those of other people, they are nonetheless amazing and distinctive in their own way.

CHAPTER 4

AFFECTED POPULACE

The Ehlers-Danlos syndrome is a complex condition that manifests itself in a wide variety of various ways throughout the body. As a direct consequence of this, individuals who are affected by this illness may be identified from others in a number of different ways.

A Community Comprised Of Many Facets Bound Together By A Common Allegiance

There is a very small population of people that live in this very unique setting, and these people all have one thing in common: they all have Ehlers-Danlos Syndrome. There is no minimum or maximum age requirement to participate in this forum debate.

It is not impossible for it to have an effect on the lives of people of all ages, including newborns, children, adolescents, and adults. In this one-of-a-kind civilization, there are no restrictions placed on anybody based on their gender, and people of either gender are encouraged to take part in the activities.

The Ehlers-Danlos Syndrome is analogous to a strange enigma that might unexpectedly present itself in the body of any individual.

The Effects Of Eds On The Human Body Are Exposed, Revealing A Long-Held Mystery

When it comes to some individuals, the joints in their body seem to have an incredible potential for stretching, quite similar to that of rubber bands. There is a catch to these people's incredible flexibility, despite the fact that they may seem to have a miraculous level of control over their bodies.

In the same way that overstretching a rubber band may cause it to snap, the joints in their bodies are also susceptible to damage if they are stretched beyond their normal range of motion, especially when they are young. Living with Ehlers-Danlos disease has a number of obstacles, one of the most significant of which is attempting to strike a balance between being open and being prudent.

It's possible that Ehlers-Danlos syndrome will also leave its mark on the skin, which is the body's most visible organ and acts as its primary barrier against the environment.

The skin of some individuals who have Ehlers-Danlos syndrome is very elastic, but the skin of other people with the condition is not as stretchy as the first group's. However, if the skin is not properly cared for, its flexibility may cause it to become delicate and more prone to tearing.

People who have Ehlers-Danlos syndrome often have to take extra care to protect their skin from ripping and other issues that might arise as a result of the condition.

The motion and function of our bodies are controlled by our skeletal muscles, which are sometimes referred to as the "engines" of our mobility. Having Ehlers-Danlos Syndrome, on the other hand, may result in these engines having far less power than they should have for some individuals.

People who have this illness could notice that their muscles tire more rapidly than normal, or that certain tasks are more difficult for them to do.

In spite of this, they make it a point to participate in the activities they like in a manner that is determined as well as innovative.

Support Networks: Medical Professionals, Mental Health Professionals And Self-Care.

In the context of Ehlers-Danlos syndrome, the function of physicians is analogous to that of private investigators. They look into the aspects that go into the creation of these one-of-a-kind persons and research how Ehlers-Danlos Syndrome manifests itself physically in the bodies of those who are afflicted by it.

Those who have Ehlers-Danlos condition may have a better awareness of the signals that their bodies are providing them with their assistance, and they may be better able to tackle the challenges that are presented by the condition.

The therapist's job is comparable to that of a coach or teacher in that they guide patients through exercises and procedures that are intended to increase their level of physical fitness. People who have Ehlers-Danlos syndrome work with therapists to build their muscle strength and joint stability, in a manner that is analogous to the way athletes work with coaches to improve their skills.

Participation in self-care techniques may be of tremendous value to those who are diagnosed with Ehlers-Danlos syndrome. People who have Ehlers-Danlos syndrome often create their own instruction manuals using the knowledge they have gained about their medical condition. These manuals are based on the information they have collected.

As a consequence of having access to this knowledge, they are thus in a position to take responsibility for their health and to make choices that are advantageous to it.

The Highs And Lows Of Living With EDS On A Day-To-Day Basis

Every day has its own one-of-a-kind set of obstacles and possibilities for achievement. Those who have Ehlers-Danlos syndrome are required to make adjustments to their way of life so that they may fulfill the unique criteria that are associated with their disease.

Altering their level of physical activity and making healthier food choices are two examples of these changes that may be necessary.

Even while Ehlers-Danlos Syndrome affects a number of different parts of the body, it does not, in any way, define an individual's whole existence. People who with Ehlers-Danlos syndrome are nevertheless able to follow their passions, develop meaningful relationships, and make significant contributions to the communities in which they reside.

Keeping An Eye On And Respecting Each Person's Uniqueness Via EDS And Personal Identity

It is crucial to bear in mind that their identity is not only constituted of their sickness, despite the fact that Ehlers-Danlos Syndrome may differentiate them physically. This is because their disease is just one component of their identity.

They are balancing being students, artists, and friends while still attempting to realize their goals and realize their aspirations. They, just like everyone else, have aspirations and objectives for the years to come.

CHAPTER 5

CORRELATED CONDITIONS

Associated illnesses are analogous to companions that accompany Ehlers-Danlos Syndrome on its winding path, and when taken together, they provide an in-depth understanding of the challenges that individuals who have Ehlers-Danlos Syndrome face in their day-to-day lives.

A Complex Network Of Interconnected Causes And Effects

Certain illnesses often coexist with Ehlers-Danlos Syndrome, and the manner in which they interact with one another may have a substantial influence on the lives of persons who are plagued by both of these conditions.

One of the most common conditions that are related with this is called hypermobility. On the other hand, persons diagnosed with Ehlers-Danlos syndrome may have hinges that are not as sturdy as the average person's.

This flexibility may lead to a condition known as hypermobility, which is a state in which the joints are able to move farther than they typically would. It would be the same as allowing the door to swing open too far if it were left unlocked.

Those that are blessed with this ability also face a difficult challenge as a result of it. Extreme caution is necessary, however, both to protect one's joints and to enable astonishing feats like bending one's fingers backwards without risking injury.

Pain, which is another condition that is related with Ehlers-Danlos Syndrome, may be similar to a shadow that follows those who have the ailment and are affected by it. Imagine that you have a pebble the size of a pin lodged inside of one of your shoes.

It doesn't matter how little it is; even if it's not very big, it might still cause a substantial amount of discomfort. Those who have Ehlers-Danlos syndrome may also have pain in their muscles, joints, and even their skin at certain points during their lives.

Another problem that might arise is as a result of being very tired. Imagine that your body is a battery that delivers the power for all of your activities. Think of it like this. It is probable that someone who has Ehlers-Danlos syndrome will go through this battery far more quickly than the average person would.

Imagine you are racing in a race, and just before you cross the finish line, you start to feel your energy level drop. Those who have Ehlers-Danlos Syndrome can use this phrase to explain how exhausted they feel when they have it. It's the same as having a battery that has to be recharged at regular intervals throughout the day.

Joint Problems: Beyond Hypermobility

In certain people with Ehlers-Danlos syndrome, dislocations of the joints are a possible consequence of the condition. This might potentially be rather unpleasant, and in order to put things back in order, you will need to seek professional medical care.

People who have Ehlers-Danlos syndrome may need the use of braces or other supports to aid in maintaining the stability of their joints. Braces and other supports may be purchased from medical supply stores. Adding extra pieces to a jigsaw puzzle in order to make it more stable is an analogy for what is happening here.

The Heart Of The Matter: Cardiac Concerns

People with certain forms of Ehlers-Danlos syndrome may have some minor differences in the way that this clock operates. It is the same as having a clock that ticks at random intervals either too rapidly or too slowly, depending on the circumstance.

Ehlers-Danlos syndrome has the potential to have a detrimental effect on both the anatomy and function of the heart, which may result in cardiac issues that need strict monitoring.

One of the most significant conditions that are related with it is called Postural Orthostatic Tachycardia Syndrome, or POTS for short. Just for a moment, try to picture yourself trying to get up all of a sudden and feeling as if you are about to pass out.

It's probable that folks who have POTS find themselves going through this rather often. It's possible that this might bring on symptoms like dizziness, a speeding heartbeat, and even passing out in really unusual circumstances.

The Ehlers-Danlos Syndrome And Its Impact On Mental Health The Powerful Fighters

People who have Ehlers-Danlos syndrome could struggle with their mental health, which is one of the challenges associated with the condition. Those who have Ehlers-Danlos syndrome may at times have more difficulty along their journey due to mental health difficulties.

People who have Ehlers-Danlos Syndrome may have mental health issues such as anxiety and depression, much like clouds after a rainstorm. They are more likely to have frequent experiences of anxiousness and melancholy. Because of the challenges they are experiencing with their mental health, which may have a detrimental effect on their overall welfare, they need the support and understanding of their family, friends, and medical professionals.

Mysteries Of The Digestive System And The Lies We Tell Ourselves About Our Skin

If you have Ehlers-Danlos Syndrome, this treasure box may contain a digestive problem that is not immediately obvious. People who suffer from Ehlers-Danlos Syndrome may have digestive issues, which may be compared to having a picky treasure box that needs special attention.

Patients who have Ehlers-Danlos syndrome may have a variety of skin-related symptoms, the most common of which is a reduction in the skin's natural suppleness. People who have EDS often have skin that is very sensitive. It is quite necessary to ensure that their skin continues to be happy and healthy.

Through The Lens Of "Putting It All Together," Gaining An Understanding Of The Complicated Nature Of Correlations

Every related condition is like a thread in a tapestry; it weaves its own particular story into the very fabric of their existence. Disorders affecting the joints, the heart, the digestive system, the intellect, and the skin, are in addition to sensitivity to certain foods and substances.

All of these pieces of the jigsaw fit together to make the one-of-a-kind experiences that individual who have Ehlers-Danlos syndrome go through throughout their lives.

Finding Your Way Through EDS And All Of Its Correlations While Exploring The Benefits Of Compatibility

People who have Ehlers-Danlos syndrome are able to continue navigating the rivers of life with bravery, persistence, and the strength that comes from the power that comes from the power of unity when they have support, understanding, and resilience.

CHAPTER 6

ASSOCIATED DISORDER

Ehlers-Danlos Syndrome (EDS), a severe ailment that damages connective tissues, often travels with a few traveling companions, which are referred to as associated disorders. Together, these conditions are referred to as EDS's "traveling companions."

Those who suffer from Ehlers-Danlos Syndrome and any of the ailments that are associated with it go through life together and, as a consequence, their lives are molded by the experience.

The Complicated Network Of Ailments That Are Linked To One Another

There is a disorder known as dysautonomia that is closely associated with it. Dysautonomia is a disorder that has been likened to a button that is too sensitive because it does not always respond in the proper manner. As a consequence of this, changes may occur in a variety of body systems, including the pace of the heart, blood pressure, and even digestion.

Mast cell activation syndrome, more often referred to as MCAS, is another condition that will accompany you on your journey. When it comes to those who have MCAS, these safety precautions could at times be a bit too watchful than necessary.

It would be the same as having security staff who would sound the alarm even when there was no danger to the building. This might lead to symptoms such as allergies, digestive difficulties, or even skin problems.

A Look at Orthostatic Intolerance and Postural Orthostatic Tachycardia Syndrome in Greater Detail

Orthostatic intolerance (OI) may be broken down into many subtypes, one of which being postural orthostatic tachycardia syndrome (often known as POTS). People who have POTS may experience these symptoms even when they are not engaging in any physical activity. It's almost as if the person's heart begins racing for no apparent cause at all.

It's possible that this might bring on symptoms like dizziness, a speeding heartbeat, and even passing out in really unusual circumstances.

Symptoms Of The Digestive System Examined Through The Looking Glass

There is a possibility that conditions such as gastroesophageal reflux disease (GERD) are analogous to a smoldering fire that is confined inside their bodies. Two symptoms that may be produced by gastroesophageal reflux disease (GERD) include heartburn and the feeling that there is a fire burning in the chest.

Maintaining A Positive Mental Attitude: Ehlers-Danlos Syndrome And Mental Health

People who have Ehlers-Danlos Syndrome may have mental health concerns that are substantially analogous to those thorns. It is essential that they take care of their mental health on their journey since there is a risk that they could encounter mental health disorders such as anxiety and depression while they are away.

CHAPTER 7

ROOT CAUSES

An examination of the underlying factors that contribute to the development of this difficult illness, which shows itself in the connective tissues of the body, is required in order to meet the requirement.

During the course of this inquiry, we will look at the genetic underpinnings, the important role that collagen plays, as well as the intricate jigsaw pieces that combine to produce the one-of-a-kind tapestry that is Ehlers-Danlos Syndrome.

Bringing To Light The Mysteries Of The Genetic Nexus And Investigating The Origins Of Eds

The scribbles, which are recorded as a code in your DNA, serve as a blueprint for your whole life. They determine everything from your physical appearance to your personality. The Ehlers-Danlos Syndrome, on the other hand, adds some unexpected curves and turns to an otherwise straightforward piece of music.

These mutations are the genetic underpinnings of Ehlers-Danlos syndrome, and it is crucial to acquiring knowledge of the illness that we shed light on the functions that they play in the syndrome.

One way of looking at the many Ehlers-Danlos syndrome subtypes is as if they each relate to a distinct chapter in the larger genetic narrative. Some of the chapters have much more substantial deviations from the norm than the others.

The Most Important Role That Collagen Plays Is In Constructing The Framework Of The Body.

Collagen serves as the foundation that binds everything together, including soft skin, flexible joints, and sturdy blood vessels. Additionally important in the development of blood vessels is the protein collagen.

Patients who have been diagnosed with Ehlers-Danlos Syndrome have an abnormality in their collagen, which is the piece of the jigsaw that doesn't quite fit correctly. The consistency of the whole system is called into question as a direct result of this difference.

In a similar fashion, Ehlers-Danlos Syndrome is caused by collagen that is either weaker or poorly formed, which leads in the manifestation of the symptoms that are distinctive of the illness.

A Holistic Point Of View On Education: Finding The Missing Pieces Of The Puzzle

It is possible to draw parallels between the modification of genetic codes and the creation of jigsaw pieces that deviate from the standard. These variations are the cause of the changes that take place in the structure and function of the organism. These genetic variants have a substantial effect on the lives of individuals who have Ehlers-Danlos syndrome, just as the pieces that are missing from a jigsaw puzzle cause the entire thing to seem incomplete.

The presence of collagen anomalies adds a new dimension to the overall image. Because of these abnormalities, the connective tissues become more brittle, which, in turn, finally leads in the traits and consequences that are diagnostic of Ehlers-Danlos syndrome.

A Conglomeration Of Influencing Factors Comprising The Complexity Of Genetics

Picture a symphony being performed by an orchestra, with each individual instrument contributing its own unique tune to the overall composition. This concept is shown by the Ehlers-Danlos syndrome, which may be seen as a genetic symphony since the individual genes and all of the different permutations of those genes join together to produce the condition as a whole. This notion can be seen mirrored in the syndrome's name, which derives from the Greek words for "elastic" and "danlos," respectively.

The Ehlers-Danlos syndrome is not generated by a single defective gene but rather by the complicated interaction of numerous genes that are involved in the regulation of connective tissue function. This interaction can only occur in people who have a family history of the condition. In a way somewhat unlike to that described above, the manifestation of various Ehlers-Danlos syndrome subtypes is caused by the interplay of a number of genes.

An Enigma That Is Made Up Of A Number Of Different Factors, Including Environmental And Other Influences

It is possible for variables other than a person's genetic coding to influence the expression of Ehlers-Danlos Syndrome. These factors include environmental factors and other features of a person's surrounding environment.

Environmental influences operate as the light that sheds insight into this riddle by generating changes in the behavior of the many components that make up the genetic code. Ehlers-Danlos Syndrome is a genetic disorder that may appear in the body in a variety of different ways.

The manner in which it does so depends on a number of environmental factors that interact with the genetic framework. Nutrition, physical exercise, and mental and emotional stress are all included in these criteria.

CHAPTER 8

PREVENTIVE STRATEGIES

To ensure that certain delicate threads in the intricate tapestry that is health and well-being are resilient and strong, the weaving of those threads requires a great deal of care and attention to detail. Ehlers-Danlos Syndrome (EDS), a complex genetic disorder that affects connective tissues, compels us to examine the realm of preventive techniques.

The Primary Goal Of Early Intervention Is To Foster Resiliency From The Very Beginning.

The process of early intervention for Ehlers-Danlos syndrome operates in a way that is comparable to that which was discussed above. Its main purpose is to identify and address problems in order to prevent such issues from escalating into more significant concerns.

Early intervention in Ehlers-Danlos syndrome helps to lessen the likelihood of experiencing challenges, analogous to the way that tending to a garden prevents weeds from taking over the whole area.

Early diagnosis of Ehlers-Danlos syndrome is equivalent to early identification of the ailment. Early diagnosis of Ehlers-Danlos syndrome is similar to discovering the first buds of a flower. In circumstances involving children, the presence of certain symptoms, including joint hypermobility, skin elasticity, and developmental delays, may be markers of a possible issue.

Early intervention may take many forms, including physical therapy and monitoring of the patient's cardiac health. It begins when these warning symptoms prompt medical personnel to examine more closely at the patient's condition.

The Power Of Knowledge: The Crucial Part That Education Plays In Serving As A Preventative Measure

In the context of Ehlers-Danlos syndrome, education serves as a map that directs individuals, caregivers, and healthcare professionals down the route toward prevention. When people have access to information, they are better equipped to navigate potential roadblocks and make decisions based on the knowledge they have.

A greater awareness of Ehlers-Danlos syndrome in a community might be compared to installing signposts along a route to spread information. When individuals learn more about a disease, they become more aware of the signs of that disease, and they are also more inclined to seek medical care when it is required to do so. In a similar vein, medical practitioners who are well-informed are better equipped to detect Ehlers-Danlos syndrome in its early phases and provide patients advice on preventive measures that are individually suited to fit their needs.

Making adjustments to your way of life in order to enhance your body's resilience People who have Ehlers-Danlos Syndrome may be able to strengthen their body's resilience by making adjustments to their way of life, which is equivalent to enhancing the sturdiness of a bridge so that it can survive a number of different stressors. It is of the highest significance to engage in physical activity that will result in the growth of muscles, the provision of support for joints, and the promotion of cardiovascular health.

The job of a physical therapist, which may be likened to the labor of a mason in the construction of a bridge, plays an essential role in the process of increasing overall mobility and strengthening weak sections of the body.

Consider the building of the bridge: it is possible to protect the joints from strain and the danger of dislocation by strengthening them via the use of the appropriate workouts and activities. This might prevent the joints from being dislocated.

The Importance Of Proper Nutrition In The Maintenance And Improvement Of One's Health And Well-Being

Those who suffer from Ehlers-Danlos Syndrome will find that acquiring the proper nutrition is analogous to having a fertile field to develop on since it not only feeds the body but also helps to enhance vitality and overall wellness.

It is useful to strengthen the body's resistance by consuming a diet that is well-balanced and rich in a variety of vitamins, minerals, and proteins. This may be done by adopting a healthy lifestyle.

In the same way that equipment is required for the maintenance of the connective tissues of the body, the body also requires nutrients such as vitamin C, which contributes to the creation of collagen and is vital for its maintenance. People who have Ehlers-Danlos syndrome absolutely have to take the necessary precautions to ensure that their meals include an adequate quantity of essential nutrients.

The Importance Of Collaborative Care When It Comes To Overcoming Challenges Together

The treatment of Ehlers-Danlos syndrome may be accomplished via the use of a strategy known as collaborative care, which takes a multidisciplinary approach. People, therapists, and healthcare practitioners all working together as part of a team are included here.

These parts are seamless when placed inside the framework of collaborative care; there is no space between them. Mobility is a primary focus for physical therapists and mental health practitioners alike, and mental health experts provide emotional support to patients.

Hereditary and cardiovascular aspects of the illness are treated by professionals in the medical field. In the same way that different instruments in a well-balanced orchestra each contribute something distinctive to the overall symphony of care, so do each of the participants.

Enhancing One's Mental Well-Being By Way Of Improving One's Emotional Health

Maintaining mental health is equivalent to keeping that candle burning when it comes to the treatment of Ehlers-Danlos syndrome. This involves offering psychological aid to make the journey more comfortable. Treatment for mental health issues should be an integral component of any preventive measures since the challenges brought on by Ehlers-Danlos disease may sometimes throw shadows.

Professionals in the area of mental health assist people in the development of resilience and coping techniques in much the same way that a gardener helps flowers blossom through the application of care and attention. The Ehlers-Danlos syndrome is accompanied by a variety of emotional disorders, all of which are identified, treated, and regulated in order to guarantee that patients are able to traverse their health journey with the strength and a good attitude.

CHAPTER 9

DIAGNOSIS PROCESS

In the realm of health and medical study, solving the mysteries that surround certain diseases requires a tactic that is one that is rigorous as well as exhaustive. One of these mysteries is referred to as Ehlers-Danlos Syndrome or EDS for short. In order to arrive at an accurate diagnosis of EDS, it is necessary for patients as well as professionals in the medical field to navigate a complex diagnostic road.

The First Assessment Is Represented By An All-Encompassing Clinical Canvas.

The first evaluation for the purpose of identifying Ehlers-Danlos syndrome is akin to a blank canvas in terms of the diagnostic procedure. On this canvas, medical practitioners will begin to paint a picture of an individual's progress through their own health as they go through their life. As part of this examination, we are going to perform a comprehensive inquiry into the patient's medical history, as well as their symptoms and physical traits.

In the same way that an artist takes great care in selecting their brushstrokes and colors, medical practitioners take great care in putting together the parts of the medical jigsaw puzzle that pertains to the patient. They inquire about symptoms such as frequent dislocations of the joints, hypermobility of the joints, and elasticity of the skin. This information acts as the first strokes on the canvas of being aware of Ehlers-Danlos Syndrome, and it is the foundation around which the process of diagnosis is constructed.

The Significance Of Researching One's Family History In Order To Unearth Previously Unknown Genetic Connections

Gaining an awareness of one's family history is akin to untangling those threads when searching for genetic patterns that might give insights in the context of obtaining a diagnosis of Ehlers-Danlos

Syndrome. This is because both processes include looking for clues in genetic patterns.

The healthcare experts inquire with the patient's family members about whether or not they have had any symptoms that are associated with Ehlers-Danlos Syndrome. This inquiry may bring to light a genetic thread that has been handed down through generations, providing insight, as a result, into the hereditary basis of Ehlers-Danlos Syndrome.

A family tree may reveal information on the genetic origins of Ehlers-Danlos Syndrome in a specific lineage in the same way as the patterns in a tapestry may tell a story about its history.

An Inquiry Into One's Physical Selves With The Aim Of Disclosing One's Physical Blueprint

The Ehlers-Danlos syndrome may be diagnosed by a procedure that consists of a detailed assessment of the patient's physical condition. During this phase of the process, the medical experts assess the patient's physical characteristics in order to identify whether or not the patient may be afflicted by the illness.

Medical personnel will examine everything from the pliability of the skin to the hypermobility of the joints and even the surface texture of the skin itself. The medical community has described a number of physical traits that have the potential to be indicators of Ehlers-Danlos syndrome.

At this point in the diagnostic process, the joints are subjected to some light manipulation in order to assess the range of motion and flexibility available in that particular joint. This is a crucial stage in the process that must not be skipped.

How To Navigate Your Way Around Genetic Testing Using "The Genetic Path"

In the instance of Ehlers-Danlos syndrome, doing genetic testing is akin to going along these routes in an attempt to find certain genetic variations that are associated to the condition.

During genetic testing, a person's DNA is studied to look for changes in genes that are known to be connected with Ehlers-Danlos syndrome. This is done so that a diagnosis of EDS may be made. With the assistance of genetic testing, medical professionals are able to successfully cross the treacherous terrain that is an individual's genetic make-up.

This method both elucidates the genetic basis of Ehlers-Danlos syndrome and establishes the occurrence of particular gene changes that are linked with the disorder.

The Utilization Of The Collaborative Method, Which Includes Contributions From Specialists In A Wide Range Of Fields

The procedure of diagnosing Ehlers-Danlos syndrome also makes use of a collaborative approach similar to the one described above. In this method, a group of healthcare professionals from a variety of backgrounds collaborate to provide an accurate and exhaustive assessment.

Healthcare professionals from a wide array of fields, such as geneticists, orthopedic specialists, dermatologists, and cardiologists, join together to discuss their points of view. It is guaranteed that no aspect of the diagnosis procedure for Ehlers-Danlos syndrome will be ignored thanks to the involvement of specialists from a broad variety of areas in this joint effort.

How To Navigate Your Way Through The Complexity That Is Differential Diagnosis

An essential part of the process of diagnosing Ehlers-Danlos Syndrome is ruling out the presence of any other conditions that might be responsible for symptoms that are analogous to those of the syndrome itself. Utilizing this technique, also known as differential diagnosis, will always lead to the correct diagnosis being reached.

Medical specialists will rule out the likelihood that another condition is the root cause of a patient's symptoms before establishing that the patient has Ehlers-Danlos syndrome. Decisions made by healthcare practitioners are always thoroughly thought out and based on careful inspection and assessment of the relevant information. At this point, there is no longer any chance of producing an inaccurate diagnosis, which guarantees that the diagnostic technique will provide reliable results.

Obtaining A Particular Diagnosis Is Currently The Missing Link In The Chain Of Events

The technique of arriving at a definitive diagnosis of Ehlers-Danlos Syndrome is comparable to completing a challenging jigsaw puzzle; this is the stage at which all of the components of the diagnostic process come together to form a whole.

After taking into consideration the findings of a clinical evaluation, the patient's family history, a physical examination, genetic testing, and group discussions, medical practitioners are able to arrive at a diagnosis. The provision of solutions to issues that may have lingered even after other treatments or tests have been finished is one of the many ways in which a definite diagnosis may provide clarity to the individual's journey through the realm of health care.

The Role That A Person's Diagnosis Plays In Determining How Well They Can Make Informed Decisions

The provision of a person with Ehlers-Danlos Syndrome with a diagnosis serves as a lantern, offering both the individual and those who care about them with a source of light along the challenging route of treating the condition.

When a person is given a diagnosis, they have a greater understanding of their symptoms, the challenges they are experiencing, and the potential outcomes that may be in store for them.

People who have access to information are in a better position to make well-informed decisions regarding the course of their journey through the healthcare system. They are able to examine the many different therapeutic options available to them, make adjustments to the manner in which they live their lives, and connect with support networks that are tailored specifically to their need.

An accurate diagnosis of Ehlers-Danlos syndrome eliminates the need for conjecture and provides the way for proactive medical treatment, both of which contribute to an improvement in the patient's quality of life.

CHAPTER 10

THERAPEUTIC APPROACHES (TREATMENT)

When it comes to the intricate tapestry that is the state of a person's health, there are certain threads that need painstaking weaving in order to keep their strength and resilience intact. Ehlers-Danlos Syndrome (EDS), which is a complex group of hereditary diseases that affect connective tissues, presents a unique challenge that calls for an all-encompassing strategy for the therapeutic techniques that are utilized to treat it.

As we embark on this journey, we will investigate the many different therapeutic alternatives that are available to individuals who are living with Ehlers-Danlos Syndrome.

These possibilities range from pain management techniques to physical therapies. In addition, we will discuss the relevance of multidisciplinary cooperation in the process of weaving together a tapestry of wellness.

Understanding The Mechanisms That Contribute To Comfort As A Form Of Pain Management

In terms of the therapy for Ehlers-Danlos syndrome, the alleviation of discomfort is comparable to receiving a warm embrace. It alleviates the pain and suffering that often accompany the sickness, which is a respite that may be very much appreciated by the patient. The word "pain management" refers to a number of different approaches that may be taken to give relief from various types of pain, including both acute and chronic pain.

In the same way that a soft touch may relieve tension in painful muscles and joints, non-pharmacological therapies, such as physical therapy and gentle exercises, can do the same thing. Patients work side-by-side with their physical therapists to devise tailored workout plans. These plans are created with the goal of enhancing the patients' muscle strength and joint stability.

In the same way professional massage therapists employ certain methods to lessen their customers' levels of stress, physical therapists use treatments that assist the musculoskeletal system of the body.

The use of pharmacological treatments, such as analgesics and painkillers, may be utilized in order to obtain localized pain relief. When used exactly as prescribed by a medical professional, these medications facilitate the management of pain and provide a significant contribution to an overall improvement in quality of life.

The Part That Physical Therapies Play In Developing One's Own Inner Strength And Capacity For Resilience

The use of physical therapies to treat Ehlers-Danlos Syndrome is akin to providing extra support to the bridge; these treatments increase the body's capacity to tolerate the impacts of stress and are thus effective in treating the condition. Participation in therapeutic activities that have a focus on improving muscular strength, joint stability, and flexibility is vital in order to treat Ehlers-Danlos syndrome successfully.

These exercises should be undertaken on a regular basis. Individuals, in conjunction with the therapists who are treating them, devise exercise routines that are uniquely crafted to fulfill the prerequisites of their individual diseases. These exercises concentrate on problem areas and strive to enhance joint stability, which ultimately leads to more mobility and a reduced risk of joint dislocation.

The use of a pool is essential to the practice of hydrotherapy, which is also sometimes referred to as aquatic therapy. Just like a loving embrace, the buoyancy of water helps to cushion the stress that exercise has on your joints. Imagine the buoyancy of water as a warm hug.

Individuals are supplied with a low-impact environment in which to engage in exercises that develop muscles without hurting the joints while engaging in hydrotherapy sessions that are led by qualified professionals. In addition, these individuals are provided with the opportunity to interact with other individuals who are also undergoing treatment for similar conditions.

The Importance Of Establishing A Solid Foundation When Performing Orthopedic Interventions

Orthopedic therapies for Ehlers-Danlos syndrome are relatively comparable to treatments for other types of the ailment that are utilized for the same purpose. These therapies focus on stabilizing the affected joints in order to prevent further complications, such as dislocations.

Tools such as braces and splints are examples of orthopedic devices. These tools work to stabilize the joints by providing support for them. Imagine these devices as scaffolding that reinforces the structure of the body, therefore minimizing excessive movement that might potentially lead to joint instability.

This is the advantage that can be gained by using these technologies. Orthopedic specialists work closely with their patients to devise and prescribe customised medical devices that are customized to satisfy the needs that are unique to each individual patient.

Surgical procedures, which are comparable to carefully crafted works of art, are required in order to successfully cure severe joint instability. Patients diagnosed with Ehlers-Danlos syndrome who suffer from joint dislocations that happen often and cause severe handicap may have the option of undergoing surgical procedures as a potential treatment option. The surgeries that surgeons do to repair and replace injured joints provide patients with more stability and an overall improvement in their quality of life.

The Care That Is Delivered As A Result Of Collaborative Efforts Is Analogous To A Symphony Of Expertise.

When it comes to the treatment of Ehlers-Danlos syndrome, collaborative care operates in a manner somewhat unlike to that of a symphony. In this approach, medical professionals from a wide range of specialties contribute their knowledge and experience in their respective fields to the formulation of an all-encompassing treatment plan.

In order to build a multidisciplinary team, professionals from a number of professions, such as geneticists, orthopedic specialists, physical therapists, and experts in pain management, are brought together. When therapy is administered in a way that emphasizes collaboration among the many providers, it is possible to ensure that each and every aspect of an individual's sickness is addressed, from the genetic foundations to the techniques for relieving pain.

Nutritional Counseling: Promoting Internal And External Health And Well-Being From The Ground Up

Those who suffer from Ehlers-Danlos Syndrome will find that acquiring the proper nutrition is analogous to having a fertile field to develop on since it not only feeds the body but also helps to enhance vitality and overall wellness. When it comes to the maintenance of healthy connective tissue, it is of the utmost importance to consume a diet that is not only nutritionally sound but also rich in the nutrients that are of benefit to this tissue.

Vitamins, such as vitamin C, are fundamental to the process of producing collagen, which in turn serves to preserve the structural integrity of connective tissues. When people are given nutritional advice, it ensures that they will consume the essential nutrients that are necessary to maintain the health of their connective tissues as well as their overall wellbeing.

Taking Care Of One's Emotional Health And Developing Coping Mechanisms For Dealing With Stress

Because they provide patients with the skills required to navigate the emotional complexity that often accompanies the condition, the coping strategies that are utilized in the therapy of Ehlers-Danlos Syndrome are akin to that guiding hand.

When individuals take part in counseling or support groups that are conducted by professionals in the field of mental health, they are given access to a safe space in which they are able to verbalize their feelings and gain useful tools with which to deal with difficult situations. In the same way that a compass points individuals in the direction of emotional resilience and general well-being, these strategies point people in that direction.

The treatment plan for Ehlers-Danlos syndrome must always include the patient's mental health being prioritized as a central focus of attention. Patients are able to develop resiliency and a positive mindset as a result of this treatment, which helps them handle the challenges they experience.

CHAPTER 11

ALTERNATIVE TREATMENT APPROACHES

When it comes to issues concerning one's health and well-being, the approaches that have been used traditionally are often what serve as the foundation of medical therapy. Alternative treatment approaches, on the other hand, may give patients suffering from complex conditions such as Ehlers-Danlos syndrome (EDS) with a fresh entry point to pain relief and an improved quality of life.

As a first step in our inquiry, we are going to investigate the field of alternative remedies, which might include anything from acupuncture to herbal therapy. Our objective is to provide insight on how these alternative treatments could work in conjunction with conventional therapies and make a contribution to the management of Ehlers-Danlos syndrome as a whole.

Comprehending The Complementary And Alternative Medical Practices From A Holistic Perspective.

Treatments that are deemed traditional often center their attention on certain facets of the issue, and as a result, they tackle symptoms and challenges in an indirect manner. Alternative therapies, on the other hand, take a holistic approach to health care, which means that they aim to restore balance and harmony to the body as a whole rather than merely treating particular symptoms.

This is in contrast to conventional treatments, which only address the symptoms that a patient is experiencing.

Treatments that use a holistic approach, such as chiropractic care and acupuncture, adopt the philosophy that the human body may be seen as an interconnected system.

The practitioners of these therapies have as their primary objective to address the underlying imbalances that contribute to the symptoms of Ehlers-Danlos syndrome in order to restore balance and alleviate any discomfort that may be connected with the condition.

Controlling The Flow Of Energy Through The Use Of Acupuncture As An Art Form

The ancient practice of acupuncture, which goes back thousands of years, may be thought of as providing this energy flow a tiny push in the appropriate direction in order to preserve homeostasis and reduce pain. In order to promote the body's intrinsic ability for healing, acupuncture includes the insertion of extremely thin needles into key sites all over the body. These areas vary from person to person.

Acupuncturists tailor the treatment regimens they provide patients to the unique needs of each individual patient in order to reduce patients' levels of pain, increase their circulation, and otherwise enhance their general health. Those who are experiencing the symptoms that are linked with Ehlers-Danlos syndrome may find some relief if the energies inside their bodies are brought back into harmony.

Adjusting The Anatomy Of The Body Is Part Of The Care Chiropractors Provide For Patients

A chiropractic adjustment is similar to making a tweak to the foundation of something in order to make it more stable. Manual adjustments are made to patients by chiropractors in order to realign the spine and the joints, which ultimately leads to an improvement in posture and a reduction in pain.

Chiropractors conduct these adjustments on patients.

Chiropractors work closely with their patients to devise specialized treatment plans that are customized to fulfill the needs that are unique to each individual patient. By focusing on the patient's posture and alignment, chiropractic therapy assists in the preservation of healthy joints and the musculoskeletal system as a whole in the body.

Herbal Medicine Fosters A Healthy Connection With The Natural World Via Its Use Of Plants.

Herbal therapy taps on the restorative power of plants and the natural world as a whole in order to treat a diverse spectrum of medical ailments. Herbalists may suggest different plant treatments and therapies that are based on plants to their patients in the hope that these remedies would help alleviate some of the symptoms that are linked with Ehlers-Danlos Syndrome.

In the process of reducing pain and inflammation, herbs like turmeric, which is well-known for the anti-inflammatory properties that it contains, operate as natural allies. When choosing and mixing herbs in an attempt to relieve pain and enhance health, herbalists take into consideration the individual needs of each patient.

The Integration Of Mind And Body Therapies: Constructing Your Very Own Internal Strength

Meditation and other mind-body activities, such as yoga and tai chi, are analogous to ripples on the surface of the water; they promote a sense of inner peace and resilience. These practices focus an emphasis on the connection that exists between the mind and the body. In addition, they equip people with skills that may be utilized to manage stress and enhance their emotional well-being.

Through the practices of meditation, individuals have the opportunity to learn how to create awareness, which, in turn, helps to decrease tension and promote calm. On the other hand, yoga is very much like dance in the sense that it places an emphasis on flexibility and balance while also teaching gentle movement that is good for the health of the joints.

Manual Therapies: Mastering The Art Of Touching Patients To Heal Them

People who have been diagnosed with Ehlers-Danlos Syndrome may find that manual therapies like massage and myofascial release, which include the skilled use of touch, help them experience a sense of comfort.

A wide array of one-of-a-kind techniques are used by practitioners in order to ease muscle tension, enhance circulation, and give support for the proper functioning of joints.

People may enhance their flexibility and feel less pain by using a technique called myofascial release, which is a strategy that offers them with a way to reduce the amount of discomfort they feel. The fascia, the connective tissue that surrounds the muscles and acts as a barrier between them, is the objective of this therapy.

Manual therapies often adapt to the specific needs of each individual patient, so giving a tailored method for creating a state of relaxation and general well-being in the process.

Offering Help With Nutrition And Diet In Order To Foster Healthy Lifestyles And A Healthy Body

Nutritional and dietary support refers to the process of modifying one's diet in such a way as to provide the essential nutrients that are essential to the health of connective tissue as well as the overall well-being of the individual.

People who have Ehlers-Danlos Syndrome may be able to supply their bodies with the sustenance they need from the inside out by eating a diet that is both well-balanced and rich in vitamins and minerals. This may allow their bodies to function as effectively as possible.

Vitamins like vitamin C, which are necessary to the body, have a considerable influence, not only on the creation of collagen, but also on the overall health of the tissues. When people are offered support with their nutrition and food, they are given the tools and information they need to make well-informed choices that are beneficial to their health and their path toward better health.

Understanding The Importance Of Being Your Own Person And Developing Your Own Personalized Roadmap

Alternative therapies understand the value of individualization and give a customised approach that takes into consideration the different needs, limitations, and preferences of each individual patient.

Practitioners of alternative therapies collaborate closely with their patients and conduct in-depth examinations in order to get an in-depth comprehension of the patient's medical history and the treatment goals they want to achieve. In addition to the customized approach that has shown to be effective in the management of Ehlers-Danlos syndrome, the use of alternative treatments may also prove to be beneficial.

A Method That Is Characterized By Its Ability To Strike A Balance Between Collaboration And Communication

When complementary alternative treatments and conventional medical approaches are used in the management of Ehlers-Danlos syndrome, one may say that the condition has been brought to a point of balance.

In order to create a united and holistic strategy, it is vital to have productive communication and work together in order to interact successfully among individuals, healthcare experts, and alternative therapists. This is required in order to ensure that an approach is taken that is well-rounded

CHAPTER 12

IDEAL DIET FOR MANAGING EHLERS-DANLOS SYNDROME

When it comes to a person's overall health and sense of well-being, the significance of eating a balanced and nutritious diet cannot be overstated. Those who are living with the challenges of Ehlers-Danlos Syndrome (EDS) are in a position where nutrition takes on a much more important role.

When we begin our inquiry, we will delve into the complexity of an ideal diet that is suitable for treating Ehlers-Danlos Syndrome. our diet is optimal since it is tailored to alleviate the symptoms of EDS. We will investigate the role that diet, hydration, and eating mindfully play in the formation of well-being as well as the capacity for resiliency.

The Nutritional Blueprint: Building A Stable Foundation For Your Health And Well-Being

A diet that is suitable for treating Ehlers-Danlos Syndrome is comparable to a plan that has been meticulously created. Its purpose is to facilitate the maintenance of healthy connective tissue, the regulation of inflammatory processes, and overall wellness.

Vitamins and minerals of vital importance

The production of collagen, the upkeep of healthy bones, and the regeneration of injured tissue are all processes that are considerably facilitated by the consumption of certain vitamins and minerals.

You provide your body with the building blocks it needs to function at its maximum level and ensure that it will continue to do so when you consume foods that are rich in nutrients. This enables your body to perform at its peak level.

Some Foods That Can Help Reduce Pain And Inflammation

Think of foods that are anti-inflammatory as being similar to shields that protect your body from the assault of inflammation that it is subjected to. It is likely that Ehlers-Danlos syndrome may go hand in side with chronic inflammation, which will only make the symptoms worse. If this is the case, it will only serve to exacerbate the condition.

Incorporating foods strong in antioxidants, such as colorful fruits and vegetables, as well as omega-3 fatty acids, which may be found in fatty fish and flaxseeds, helps combat inflammation and stimulates the body's natural capacity to recuperate. Some examples of foods high in antioxidants include: fruits and vegetables with bright colors.

A level or condition of hydration

It is essential that you stay properly hydrated since doing so enables you to preserve joint mobility, enhance circulation, and boost your overall vitality; so, it is imperative that you do so.

You should make it a goal to consume the recommended amount of water throughout the day, and you should also give some thought to the possibility of integrating other foods and beverages in your diet, such as watermelon, cucumbers, and herbal teas.

The Development Of A Harmonious Connection With One's Food Via The Intentional Cultivation Of Mindful Eating Practices.

The process of practicing mindful eating, which is equivalent to enjoying each individual morsel of food, may help to develop a closer connection between your body and the food that you consume. This technique is particularly useful for those who have Ehlers-Danlos syndrome since it encourages cognitive decision-making and aids to the preservation of intestinal health.

When you are eating, it is important to use all of your senses, as well as pay attention to the cues that tell you when you are hungry and when you have had enough to eat. It is essential to chew food thoroughly in order to not only make digestion easier but also to cultivate a sense of gratitude for the nutrients that are offered by the food that one consumes.

Collagen-Rich Foods That Are Beneficial To Connective Tissue Foods That Are Rich In Collagen

Comparable to the raw materials that are used in the construction process are foods that encourage the body to produce more collagen. Consuming foods like citrus fruits, bell peppers, and broccoli that are rich in vitamin C can contribute to the formation of collagen in the body.

In a similar fashion, meals that are rich in amino acids such as proline and glycine, which may be found in bone broth and other kinds of lean protein, contribute to the body's efforts to manufacture collagen.

When you include these foods in your diet, you provide your body the resources it needs to maintain the structural integrity of its connective tissues, joints, and skin. These aids include certain nutrients, such as vitamins and minerals.

Consuming Foods Known For Their Anti-Inflammatory Effects Is A Useful Strategy For Managing Inflammation.

Anti-inflammatory foods are like buckets of water that put out a fire. They reduce pain and nurture the body's capacity to heal from an injury or illness. It is extremely important to have the inflammation under control in order to improve one's general health when it comes to controlling Ehlers-Danlos syndrome.

Include in your diet foods that are strong in antioxidants, such as tomatoes, berries, and greens that are leafy, such as spinach and leafy greens. It is advised that one include into their diet foods that are high in omega-3 fatty acids, such as fatty fish (salmon, mackerel, and sardines), as well as chia seeds, in order to manage inflammatory responses and preserve healthy joints.

Hydration Is The Process Of Supplying The Needs Of The Body With Water In Order To Maintain A State Of Equilibrium.

People who have Ehlers-Danlos syndrome really must drink enough water on a daily basis in order to keep their joints lubricated, their circulation going, and their overall health in good shape.

You should make it a point to consume the necessary quantity of water throughout the day, and you should also think about eating hydrating foods like watermelon and cucumber and drinking herbal teas. Set a goal for yourself to drink the appropriate amount of water throughout the day.

Keeping a healthy level of hydration is comparable to providing your body with the essential fuel it requires in order for it to operate at its absolute peak level of performance.

While Appreciating Every Nourishing Moment That Passes While Mindfully Consuming Food

Because it helps you to fully engage in each pleasurable moment that you are eating, practicing mindful eating is analogous to creating a sacred space for your relationship with food. This is because it enables you to experience the full satisfaction that comes from eating.

Through the cultivation of the practice of mindful eating, you may be able to establish a more deep connection with the food needs and preferences of your body.

In The Wellness Symphony, The Role Of Nutritional Balance As An Instrument

The most effective way to cure Ehlers-Danlos Syndrome is to follow a diet that incorporates a broad variety of foods. These meals should not only cater to the particular requirements of your body, but should also promote your overall health and vitality.

Be sure to consume a sufficient amount of lean proteins like fish, poultry, lentils, and tofu in order to preserve the health of your muscles. Whole grains are a good source of sustained energy, and fruits and vegetables that are rich in color are filled with a broad array of vitamins, minerals, and antioxidants.

Whole grains may be found in a number of different foods. If you want to keep the lubrication in your joints and enhance your overall health, you should make sure that your diet contains healthy fats from sources such as avocados, almonds, and olive oil.

The Strength Of A Person's Resistance May Be Traced Back To The Support That Is Offered By Connective Tissue.

The support offered by connective tissue is akin to a scaffold in that it is what holds this masterpiece together while also assuring its endurance and stability. This support also ensures that the masterpiece will not fall apart. By include foods in your diet that are helpful to the health of the connective tissues, you may provide your body with the nutrients it needs to maintain its structure and ensure that it continues to function properly.

Consuming foods that are strong in vitamin C, such as citrus fruits, strawberries, and bell peppers, may help improve the body's natural synthesis of collagen. Foods that are high in sulfur, such as garlic, onions, and cruciferous vegetables, may help the body produce collagen and speed the repair of damaged tissue. Sulfur also plays a role in the production of new collagen molecules.

Extinguishing The Fires Within, Also Known As The Management Of Inflammation

The management of inflammation is akin to guiding those waves in order to restore calmness inside of your body. Patients diagnosed with Ehlers-Danlos Syndrome must have their inflammation well managed as part of their therapy in order to see a reduction in the intensity of their symptoms and an improvement in their overall health.

The Act Of Hydrating Oneself, Also Known As Replenishing The Terrain Of The Body

Those who have Ehlers-Danlos syndrome should make sure to have a healthy level of water in their bodies at all times since this helps to keep joint lubrication intact in addition to supporting general body functions.

You should make it a goal to consume the necessary amount of water each day, and you should also give some thought to the possibility of having foods and beverages in your diet that might assist you in being hydrated. Some examples of such foods and beverages are cucumbers, watermelon, and herbal teas.

Making sure that your body gets the right quantity of water each day may help you feel more energized and improve your overall health and well-being.

The Act Of Paying Attention To One's Diet As A Kind Of Preventative Self-Care

Eating in a way that is mindful is analogous to executing a ritual as a part of one's routine for the purpose of providing for one's own self-care, with each mouthful acting as a chance to express gratitude and one's objectives. This practice is beneficial for those who have Ehlers-Danlos syndrome because it teaches people to make choices in a thoughtful manner and it enhances the health of the digestive system.

You should get ready for each meal with a mindset of gratitude, and you should make use of all of your senses when you are really eating. It is essential to chew every bite of your food thoroughly in order to provide your body with the necessary nutrients and to facilitate digestion.

Eating one's meals in a thoughtful way may help to cultivate a more concordant relationship with one's diet, which in turn can improve one's overall sense of well-being.

A Healthy, Well-Balanced Diet Is The Conductor Of The Wellness Symphony.

A diet that includes a broad range of foods, each of which provides a distinct contribution to the overall harmony of one's health, would be the best way to cure Ehlers-Danlos Syndrome. Such a diet would contain a lot of different kinds of foods.

Including lean proteins in your diet, such as those that are found in fish, poultry, and lentils, may assist in the maintenance of good muscle. Whole grains are a wonderful source of prolonged energy, and fruits and vegetables that are rich in color are excellent sources of an abundance of vitamins, minerals, and antioxidants.

Whole grains also provide a good source of maintained energy. Consuming good fats such as those found in avocados, almonds, and olive oil may help increase the vitality of the joints and the body as a whole. This effect may also have a positive effect on the immune system.

Taking A Tailored Approach: Establishing Your Own Personal Nutritional Routine

The procedure of building a personalized approach to nutrition is akin to the process of tailoring one's diet to the particular needs and preferences of one's body. While general guidelines could be of some use, it is of much more significance to be aware of how your body responds to certain foods and to base your selections on this information.

Keeping a food journal can enable you to keep track of how specific meals affect not just your symptoms but also your overall health. By fine-tuning your diet based on personal observations and utilizing those to guide you, you may be able to establish a nutritional path that is supportive of your journey with Ehlers-Danlos Syndrome.

Care In Partnership: Including Counseling On The Patient's Nutritional Requirements

When it comes to the management of Ehlers-Danlos syndrome, collaborative care means includes dietary counseling as one of the tools in your toolkit. This makes it easier to verify that the decisions you make about your diet are congruent with the treatment approach you have developed as a whole.

Have a conversation with your healthcare practitioner about the foods you choose to eat, any dietary restrictions you may have, as well as any observations you've made.

When you make nutritional counseling an essential component of your overarching management approach, you generate a holistic plan that, in a variety of ways, helps to your overall health and sense of well-being.

CHAPTER 13

FOODS TO STEER CLEAR OF

When considering the intricate network of elements that influence an individual's health and well-being, it is impossible to overstate the significance of food. Foods that have the potential to worsen symptoms and create discomfort are something that individuals who live with Ehlers-Danlos Syndrome (EDS) need to be aware of. This is of the highest significance.

During the course of this inquiry, we will delve into the realm of foods that should be avoided. Our goal is to shed light on the ways in which particular dietary choices may either help or hinder the road toward curing Ehlers-Danlos Syndrome.

Taking Into Account The Fact That Every Single Person Has Their Own Unique Sensitivity Spectrum

Foods that make one person's symptoms worse may be easily tolerated by another person afflicted with the same ailment who does not have that person's condition. When it comes to decisions about one's diet, the sensitivity spectrum lays an emphasis on the relevance of individual differences in preferences and sensitivities.

Some individuals may have symptoms after eating certain meals, whilst other others may not be influenced in any way by the items in question. You will have the capacity to make informed judgments that are in keeping with your general health and wellbeing if you are aware of the specific ways in which your body responds to the many different types of food that you consume.

Identifying The Potential Causes Of Inflammation And The Foods That Trigger It

Foods that operate as inflammatory triggers are similar to gasoline in that they fuel this spark, which in turn causes the symptoms of Ehlers-Danlos Syndrome to grow more severe in people who have the condition. If you wish to reduce inflammation and make overall improvements to your health, it is imperative that you abstain from consuming the items listed above.

These meals often include a significant quantity of carbohydrates that have been processed, fats that aren't beneficial to your health, and additives. Avoid eating items that are known to cause inflammation in the body.

Some examples of these foods are processed meals, sugary snacks, and trans fats, which may be found in fried and packaged foods. These are some excellent examples of variables that might cause inflammation.

A Greater Understanding Of The Role That The Microbiome Plays In Ensuring Digestive Health

Certain foods disrupt this delicate balance, which has an impact on the health of the gut and may cause symptoms for individuals who have Ehlers-Danlos Syndrome to become more severe. It is very necessary to take care of one's stomach in order to keep inflammation under control and to guarantee that digestion is carried out correctly.

Foods that are high in refined sugars, artificial sweeteners, and excessive levels of caffeine are all examples of foods that contribute to an unhealthy environment in the stomach. Other examples include foods that are high in fat and cholesterol. It has been shown that these meals may disrupt the normal balance of bacteria that is found in the stomach, which can result in pain in the digestive tract.

Keeping Yourself Hydrated While Being Mindful Of The Choices You Make About Your Drinking

Drinks are also an essential aspect of the treatment of symptoms related with Ehlers-Danlos syndrome, despite the fact that substantial meals are often the focus of attention when it comes to this topic. Making conscientious choices about how much water and other liquids one consumes on a daily basis may have a positive impact on one's overall health and well-being if those choices are put into practice.

Because sugary beverages like soda and energy drinks have the potential to produce inflammation and a spike in blood sugar, it is best to limit your use of these drinks as much as possible. Additionally, ingesting an excessive quantity of caffeine via drinks such as coffee and some kinds of tea may disrupt regular sleep patterns and could make symptoms worse.

Caffeine can be found in a variety of foods and beverages.

Dietary Triggers For Sensitivity And Allergy Are Discussed In "Discovering Sensitivities And Allergens," Which May Be Found Here.

Sensitivities and allergies may be regarded of as signs that lead to specific dietary triggers that make symptoms worse for those who have Ehlers-Danlos syndrome. Recognizing and avoiding the presence of these triggers are both essential components of the management of one's overall health.

Gluten and dairy are two examples of typical triggers; both of these foods have the potential to cause discomfort and inflammation in the digestive system. People who have Ehlers-Danlos Syndrome may have a heightened sensitivity to certain foods, such as nightshades (which include tomatoes, eggplants, and peppers), which may exacerbate the pain and inflammation that is already present in the body.

Respecting The Signals That Your Body Sends You In Order To Eat Things In A Thoughtful Manner

Consuming food in a mindful manner is akin to actively engaging in this discussion in that one must pay close attention to the way in which varied meals influence one's body in order to consume food in a mindful manner. If you participate in this exercise, you will develop the capacity to make choices that are beneficial to your wellbeing and give you the confidence to act upon those choices.

If you find that certain foods consistently cause discomfort or make symptoms worse, you may want to consider reducing your consumption of such items or perhaps eliminating them entirely from your diet. Your journey toward Ehlers-Danlos syndrome management will be facilitated if you place your trust in the signals that your body gives you and make the necessary adjustments to the foods that you eat.

The Potential Of Subtraction: Tailoring Your Diet To Meet Your Specific Requirements

The empowerment of elimination refers to the practice of removing potential triggers from one's diet in order to observe how the body responds to the new diet. This strategy helps you to identify meals that may be contributing to the aggravation of symptoms and enables you to make informed selections that encourage feelings of comfort in a manner that is beneficial to you.

To begin, you should give up any meals that have the potential to be an allergen trigger for a certain period of time, such as two weeks to four weeks. You should ease back into eating each of these things, one at a time, while keeping a close watch on how your body responds to each new food. You will have acquired substantial insight into the manner in which different meals effect your health if your symptoms develop worse when you eat the meal again after giving it a try and seeing whether it makes a difference.

You will have the flexibility to change your food in order to meet the precise needs that your body has when you use this strategy.

Putting An End To The Mysteries Surrounding Processed Foods And Their Repercussions

People who have Ehlers-Danlos Syndrome may experience an exacerbation of their symptoms if they consume processed foods. These foods are equivalent to rough areas that disrupt the balance and have the potential to make symptoms worse. In order to reduce inflammation and improve one's general vitality, it is very essential to refrain from consuming any foods that have been processed.

These meals often include a high concentration of processed carbs, unhealthy fats, and additives, all of which have the potential to cause inflammation and pain throughout the body. Choose meals that are not processed and are abundant in nutrients since these kinds of foods not only improve overall health but also provide the necessary building blocks for connective tissues.

Avoiding Sugars That Have Been Refined As Well As Other Sources Of Excessive Sweetness.

Consuming meals that are high in refined sugars is analogous to putting fuel to a fire for those who have Ehlers-Danlos Syndrome since it causes both an increase in inflammation and an increase in discomfort. In order to properly manage symptoms and enhance one's general health, it is very vital to reduce the amount of refined sugars in one's diet or completely eliminate them from one's diet.

Sweets that have been processed, snacks high in sugar, and beverages with high sugar content often include refined sugars. Natural sweeteners like honey, maple syrup, and fruit are the way to go if you want to satiate your want for sweetness without exacerbating your symptoms. Other artificial sweeteners may have the opposite effect.

Avoiding Harmful Fats As Well As Trans Fats And Keeping A Safe Distance From Them

Consuming foods that are high in trans fats is analogous to having clouds in your path, since they impede your ability to make headway in managing the symptoms of Ehlers-Danlos Syndrome. It is very essential, in order to support healthy joints and overall vitality, to refrain from consuming foods that contain trans fats.

Fried foods, prepackaged snacks, and even certain baked goods may contain trans fats. It is essential to ingest sources of good fats including avocados, nuts, seeds, and olive oil in order to increase joint lubrication and overall health. Other foods that include healthy fats include olives.

Caffeine Use Should Be Done So With Mindfulness In Order To Effectively Control Symptoms.

Even though drinking coffee is something that a lot of people do on a regular basis, individuals who have Ehlers-Danlos syndrome should be very careful while doing so in order to ensure that they are effectively managing their symptoms. It is essential for your overall sense of well-being that you maintain close tabs not just on the quantity of caffeine you take but also on the way in which it is affecting your body.

Moderate use of caffeine may provide a short boost to one's energy levels; however, excessive consumption of caffeine may disrupt regular sleep patterns, lead to anxiety, and create discomfort. Moderate consumption of caffeine may provide a transient boost to one's energy levels.

Pay attention to how the caffeine affects your body, and if required, try reducing the amount you consume or altering it in some other way so that it better satisfies your requirements.

Examining The Effects Of Sugar Substitutes And Artificial Sweeteners

Even if they provide an alternative to sugar, the impact of sugar-free sweeteners on persons who have Ehlers-Danlos syndrome may be puzzling. This is despite the fact that sugar-free sweeteners do give an alternative to sugar.

It is vital, in order to make choices based on reliable information, to analyze the impact that artificial sweeteners have on the responses and symptoms of your body. This is because artificial sweeteners have been shown to cause serious health problems in certain people.

It is likely that some artificial sweeteners, when consumed by those who already have Ehlers-

Danlos syndrome, might cause the symptoms of the illness to become more severe. Consider keeping a record of how your body responds to the shift in routine and, if required, switching to natural sweeteners.

Finding Your Way Around Sensitivity When Dealing With Nightshades

Even though the items on this list are staples in the diets of many people, there is a chance that individuals who have Ehlers-Danlos disease will have an unpleasant response to them. In order to properly manage nightshade sensitivity, it is vital to first have an understanding of how your body responds to nightshades and then make adjustments based on that knowledge.

Vegetables and fruits with common names such as tomatoes, eggplants, and peppers are all members of the nightshade family. If you suspect that nightshades are adding to your discomfort, it is a good idea to monitor how your body responds to the consumption of such foods and investigate alternative potential remedies.

A Method That Puts The Focus On The Individual When Addressing Dairy And Gluten Sensitivities

It's possible that people who have been diagnosed with Ehlers-Danlos syndrome have various degrees of sensitivity to gluten and dairy products. To adopt a more customized approach, you must first discover how your body responds to various stimuli, and then utilize this information to make choices that support your health. Taking this approach allows you to play a more proactive role in your own health.

While it could be good for some individuals to reduce the amount of certain meals or even completely remove them out of their diet, other people might be able to manage just well eating such meals. Consider maintaining a log of how your body responds to different stimuli and speaking with experts in the area of medicine so that you may build a strategy that is tailored specifically to your needs.

The complicated process of treating Ehlers-Danlos Syndrome may be summed up by comparing it to carrying a compass that leads your meal choices. If you are aware of the foods you should avoid, this is equivalent to having the compass in your possession. You have the ability to give yourself the power to empower yourself to construct a dietary route that supports your comfort and well-being by first recognizing inflammatory triggers, then treating gut health, and ultimately controlling specific sensitivities.

Every decision you make has the potential to either stimulate resilience and vitality in your body or contribute to inflammation and discomfort. No matter which way you choose, you will have to deal with the repercussions.

Embracing habits of mindful eating, empowering the process of elimination, and personalizing your diet to match the individual needs of your body will allow you to navigate the terrain of culinary possibilities with knowledge and purpose.

CHAPTER 14

PHYSICAL ACTIVITIES (EXERCISES)

It is impossible to exaggerate the significance of participating in physically active activities in terms of the influence they have on an individual's health and well-being. People who live with Ehlers-Danlos Syndrome (EDS) really need to have a solid understanding of how to take part in activities that improve their strength, stability, and joint health in order to live a normal life.

As we go further in this inquiry, we will delve into the world of several types of physical activity, shedding light on the different kinds of workouts that are able to provide a beneficial contribution to the process of treating Ehlers-Danlos Syndrome.

PHYSICAL ACTIVITIES

Participating in physical activities, which may be seen of as a metaphor for fuel in this comparison, is one of the most effective ways to improve one's strength, flexibility, and general feeling of well-being. People who have Ehlers-Danlos syndrome should make it a top priority to engage in activities that are appropriate to their unique needs since these kinds of exercises assist preserve joint stability and increase the body's resilience to damage.

Incorporating the right amount of physical exercise into your day-to-day routine will help you develop a sense of control over your own health and well-being. Every single movement, whether it be mild stretching or particular strengthening exercises, is a crucial thread in the larger tapestry that is the treatment for Ehlers-Danlos Syndrome.

Recognizing The Unique Topography Of Your Own Body And Tailoring Your Exercises To Your Specific Needs

In the same way that people with Ehlers-Danlos syndrome are able to adapt to new circumstances, these individuals should make it a top priority to personalize their exercise routines so that they can meet the particular demands placed on their bodies. If you are familiar with the strengths, limitations, and pressure spots of your body, you will have a better idea of the kinds of physical activities that will be most helpful to your well-being.

Each exercise has to be adjusted so that it takes into account the participant's unique capabilities and the level of difficulty they are working at. With the help of this method, you will be able to ensure that you take part in physical activities that are beneficial to the structure of your body without putting your joints' stability at risk.

Participating In Activities With Low Impact Will Help Foster Healthy Joints

Participating in low-impact activities that enhance joint health is comparable for people with Ehlers-Danlos syndrome to getting compassionate touches on the joints. Participation in activities that reduce stress on the joints while simultaneously stimulating mobility is essential for the treatment of symptoms and the development of well-being in people who have rheumatoid arthritis.

The benefits of cardiovascular exercise may be gained by activities such as walking, swimming, and stationary cycling. These are all excellent possibilities since they do not impose an excessive burden on the joints. These workouts, in addition to boosting circulation, can enhance overall endurance and are thus very beneficial.

Building A Strong Foundation For Support Starts With Getting Your Muscles Stronger Via Resistance Training.

Strength training is akin to the use of tools in construction; these exercises buttress these pillars, which in turn enhance stability and joint integrity. Participating in targeted exercises that strengthen the muscles around sensitive joints is the single most essential thing you can do to treat the symptoms of Ehlers-Danlos syndrome.

Make it a priority to strengthen the muscle groups that support joints that are prone to instability, such as the shoulders, hips, and core. Concentrate your efforts in this area. When doing resistance training, which may be done with either tiny weights, resistance bands, or even just your own body weight, these muscles are kept active and challenged. This results in an improvement in the general joint stability.

Increasing Flexibility And Mobility While Maintaining A Flow Of Movement

Exercises that improve flexibility are analogous to gentle stretches in that they promote joint mobility and suppleness in the muscles.

Flexibility exercises may be found in many different forms. In order to effectively manage the discomfort that is often associated with Ehlers-Danlos syndrome, it is essential to participate in activities that increase flexibility.

Activities that include stretching, such as yoga, tai chi, and even simple stretching, assist develop flexibility and promote calmness at the same time. These exercises serve to cultivate a more mindful connection between the body and the breath, which, in turn, leads to an improvement in one's overall health.

Increasing Postural Awareness And Stability While Promoting Balance And Alignment

One's awareness of their own posture is comparable to the hand of an artist who strives to perfect the form of a sculpture by promoting balance and reducing strain. People who have Ehlers-Danlos syndrome should make it a top priority to take part in activities that promote postural alignment since doing so helps to preserve joint stability and minimizes the discomfort that is associated with the condition.

Pilates and other kinds of postural training concentrate an emphasis on increasing strength in the muscles that are essential for maintaining perfect posture. This helps ensure that the muscles are able to support the body in the most optimal position. These exercises put an emphasis on the stomach, back, and hip muscles, which not only serve to enhance stability but also reduce the risk of injury.

The Practice Of Mindful Movement Allows For The Integration Of Awareness Into Physical Activity.

The act of moving consciously is comparable to paying careful attention to this discourse, listening to the clues that your body offers you, and responding with thoughtfulness. It is very important for persons who have Ehlers-Danlos syndrome to exercise mindfully since doing so prevents them from overexerting themselves and minimizes the probability that they will have an injury.

Pay attention to how your body responds to the different motions, and adjust the intensity of your workout as well as the range of motion you do in accordance with this feedback. This strategy will prevent your body from being overworked beyond its capabilities and will encourage you to develop a fitness routine that can be kept up over the long term.

Utilizing The Expertise And Direction Of Trained Individuals During Physical Exercise

Employing the services of a professional, such as a physical therapist or exercise expert, to assist you in managing your exercise program is comparable to enlisting the assistance of a guide in order to navigate your way through the maze. When you engage with qualified specialists, you can be certain that your exercises will be customized to match your unique needs and will be carried out in a setting that is free of any hazards.

It's possible that a physical therapist or an exercise specialist may devise an individualized exercise plan for you that takes into consideration the unique challenges and goals that you're working toward. These professionals will make sure that you take part in activities that increase the stability of your joints, reduce the amount of discomfort that you experience, and help you get closer to receiving therapy for Ehlers-Danlos Syndrome.

The Preparation Phase And Post-Event Analysis: Putting Everything In Its Place To Ensure Success

The techniques of warming up and cooling down at the beginning and end of an effective exercise are comparable to the opening and closing acts of a great performance. Individuals who have Ehlers-Danlos syndrome should make it a top priority to add suitable warm-up and cool-down activities into their exercise routines. These exercises should be performed at the beginning and end of each workout. The body is better prepared for activity and more likely to recuperate when it follows these exercises.

Your exercise need to begin with some short, simple actions that will get your blood moving and warm up your muscles. If you do this, you will get the most out of your workout. After you've done your workout, it's a good idea to stretch out your muscles so that you may become more flexible and feel more relaxed. These routines not only make it less likely that someone would be hurt, but they also help the body recover more completely.

Pay Attention To Your Body And Recognize Its Limits And Signals By Paying Attention To Your Body

When you pay attention to your physical sensations, you are, in essence, paying attention to the cues that your partner is providing you and responding with consideration and courtesy. Participating in physical activities that are in sync with the signals and limits of your body is vital for managing the pain that is associated with Ehlers-Danlos syndrome.

It is important to remember that quality should always come before quantity, and that you should avoid pushing yourself beyond your limitations. If you pay attention to the cues that are being sent to you by your body, you may be able to make the space in which you move and operate seem more supportive and safe for you.

CHAPTER 15

GUIDANCE FOR COPING WITH THE CONDITION

The existence of Ehlers-Danlos syndrome (EDS) in a person's life brings with it a unique set of challenges, in addition to the opportunities that come along with it. It is hard to overstate the value of having guidance and answers to hand while individuals are navigating this confusing environment; this is so that they can better deal with the issues they are up against.

A Knowledge Of EDS, Understanding Being The Foundational Concept

When it comes to navigating the complexity of Ehlers-Danlos Syndrome, having a firm understanding of the disease is like having a compass in your hands. Having a solid grasp of the sickness is like having a solid hold of the illness. The first thing you should do to improve your chances of finding an effective treatment for Ehlers-Danlos syndrome is to empower yourself with knowledge on the many forms the illness may take, the symptoms it can cause, and the potential outcomes it might have.

After obtaining an understanding of the different subtypes of Ehlers-Danlos syndrome, the genetic factors that underlie each subtype, and the symptoms that are most common in each subtype, you will be in a position to make well-informed decisions about treatment, modifications to your way of life, and coping strategies. Due to the fact that you already have a solid foundation of information, you are now in a position where you can meet the challenges that Ehlers-Danlos syndrome presents with resilience and self-assurance.

Recognizing The Importance Of Self-Care And Acting In A Way That Benefits Both Your Physical And Mental Health

Taking care of your physical and mental health is analogous to tending to a garden in order to bring about an abundant crop of enjoyment. It is vital to adopt strategies of self-care that are suited to one's unique needs in order to properly manage the physical and emotional symptoms of Ehlers-Danlos syndrome. These effects may range from mild to severe.

Increasing the range of motion in your joints and inducing relaxation are two benefits that may be attained through the practice of low-impact exercises like yoga and tai chi. Make it a top priority to obtain adequate sleep so that you can aid your body in the process of recovering from whatever ails it. Participate in activities like reading, going for walks in the woods, or practicing mindfulness meditation, all of which are known to produce feelings of satisfaction and calm in those who partake in them.

By paying attention to both your physical and mental health, you have the opportunity to lay the groundwork for a foundation of well-being that will serve as a pillar of support for you as you navigate life with Ehlers-Danlos syndrome.

Building A Viable Network By Participating In Communities And Establishing Connections

The process of building a support network is related to the process of weaving a safety net because it allows you to rely on the experiences of other people who have been through circumstances that are similar to the one you are now going through. The development of connections with others who are going through the same challenges that are brought on by Ehlers-Danlos syndrome might contribute to the growth of a sense of belonging and solidarity in the affected individual.

Joining a support group for Ehlers-Danlos syndrome, whether it be in person or online, is a fantastic opportunity to create relationships with others who understand the struggles that you are going through. It is possible to foster a sense of community by engaging in conversations about coping strategies, actively listening to the experiences of one another, and offering emotional support; doing so may help alleviate feelings of isolation.

Obtaining The Opinions And Help Of Competent Professionals: Care Provided By Teams

Seeking the assistance of qualified professionals is comparable to enlisting the assistance of a guide in order to effectively navigate the challenges associated with the treatment of Ehlers-Danlos syndrome. If you collaborate with medical specialists whose area of expertise is Ehlers-Danlos Syndrome, you can certain that you will get comprehensive treatment and guidance that is tailored to your individual needs.

As a component of the treatment plan, it is recommended that you work in conjunction with a multidisciplinary team of medical professionals, such as geneticists, orthopedic specialists, physical therapists, and psychologists.

Because it takes into consideration the physiological, emotional, and mental aspects of Ehlers-Danlos syndrome, this interdisciplinary approach provides a complete and well-rounded strategy for the effective treatment of the illness.

Taking Charge Of Your Life By Planning Your Objectives And Working Towards Accomplishing Them

Setting targets that can really be accomplished is comparable to tending to a garden full of victories, regardless of how little some of those victories may seem at the time. If you make an effort to empower yourself by setting goals that are within your grasp, you will notice an improvement in both your sense of agency and your general sense of well-being.

No matter whether those goals are to increase the amount of time spent exercising each week, experiment with new coping tactics, or adjust their diet, setting goals provides one with direction and a sense of purpose, and it doesn't matter if those goals are to increase the amount of time spent exercising. Regardless of how large or little your achievements may be, you have every reason to feel pleased with yourself since they all have a positive impact on your overall well-being.

How To Navigate The Emotional Terrain Of Mindfulness And Stress Management For Better Health And Well-Being

The practices of mindfulness and stress management are comparable to lighthouses in that they provide light on the path through challenging emotional events and may be used to navigate safely. The cultivation of mindfulness practices increases one's capacity for emotional resilience and promotes well-being on a more comprehensive level.

It may be good to participate in activities such as deep breathing, meditation, and mindfulness exercises in order to keep your feeling of grounding and centering. Activities like writing and other forms of creative expression, as well as spending time in nature, may provide a healthy outlet for processing negative emotions and reducing anxiety. It's possible that engaging in these sorts of activities as part of an overall plan to manage stress may prove to be useful.

The Crucial Role That Communication And Advocacy Play In Ensuring That Your Voice Is Heard

Utilizing this megaphone to make sure that your concerns are heard and understood is equivalent to successfully articulating your needs and advocating for yourself. Self-empowerment, seen as a type of advocacy, is an essential component of effective treatment for patients diagnosed with Ehlers-Danlos disease.

Always have an open line of communication with your healthcare providers about your symptoms, concerns, and preferred methods of treatment. You should advocate for any necessary accommodations, such as specialist equipment or alterations to your living environment, in order to enhance the overall quality of your life. This may be accomplished by doing so.

When you advocate for yourself, you provide people the opportunity to recognize and address the requirements that you bring to the table. This increases the likelihood that your needs will be met.

The Crucial Part That Flexibility And Adaptability Play In Overcoming Challenges And Difficulties

An example that illustrates how to effectively traverse challenges by being flexible and adaptable is to adjust one's sails so that they correspond with the needs of the journey. Because Ehlers-Danlos syndrome might be difficult to foresee, it is essential to have a flexible mindset and come up with original answers to the challenges that arise as a result of having the condition.

You should approach these issues with an open mind, searching for inventive solutions to address the problems at hand, and altering your strategy in accordance with the findings of your search. If you accept flexibility as a virtue and make it your guiding principle, you will be able to conquer challenges with dignity and fortitude.

Pursuing Pleasure And Happiness While Attempting To Maintain An Optimistic Attitude

The quest of pleasure and a sense of fulfillment is like to taking a warm bath; you will have the sensation that your spirit is being nurtured, and your mental and emotional well-being will improve. Participating in activities that give you a sense of enjoyment, purpose, and fulfillment will not only make your life more enjoyable but will also increase your capacity to properly manage Ehlers-Danlos Syndrome.

Engage in activities and pursuits that pique your interest, spend time with the people who are important to you, and take pleasure in your pursuits. Not only may increasing your optimism and seeking out moments of pleasure increase your overall resilience in the face of adversity, but they can also enhance your emotional well-being, which is a huge advantage. Cultivating optimism and finding joy in the little things in life can assist you.

CONCLUSION

Ehlers-Danlos Syndrome (EDS) is a disorder that demands careful weaving in order to fit the odd threads that it adds to life's already colorful tapestry. As a consequence of our analysis, we have come up with essential strategies that will enable us to navigate this journey with poise and resilience.

Having a comprehension of EDS: Knowledge is a lamp that guides us toward making better choices and helps us to do so. The first step toward effective management is having a grasp of the many subtypes of Ehlers-Danlos syndrome, as well as the symptoms and treatment options associated with each subtype.

Taking Personal Responsibility for One's Health By making getting enough sleep a high priority, engaging in low-impact physical exercise, and searching out different means of relaxation, an individual may create for themselves a haven of health and happiness by taking personal responsibility for one's own health.

Developing Support: We are not going down this road by ourselves; we do have some company. Developing connections with others who also have Ehlers-Danlos Syndrome gives a network of understanding, empathy, and shared experiences, all of which may help to alleviate feelings of isolation.

Collaboration on a Professional Level On this road, the doctors, nurses, and other members of the medical community are our allies and collaborators. When working on a treatment plan for Ehlers-Danlos syndrome, it is important to collaborate with medical specialists who have extensive expertise in the subject. This will ensure that the therapy is comprehensive and covers the psychological as well as the physical aspects of the illness.

Defining Your Goals: Accomplishments, regardless of how little they may seem to be, are important milestones on the path to success. We offer ourselves the opportunity to steer our path with purpose when we provide ourselves with achievable goals, as well as when we take the time to recognize and appreciate the victories we have achieved.

As a shield would protect us from injury, the practices of mindfulness and emotional resilience methods allow us to face challenges with clarity and power, just as they would protect us from physical harm.

The power is in our voices when it comes to advocacy and the ability to adapt. We are able to overcome challenges in a manner that is both inventive and adaptable as a result of our ability to advocate for our desires and react to the shifting circumstances we are confronted with.

Embracing Joy: If you want to add more vibrant colors to the picture that is your life, one way to do so is by engaging in pursuits that provide you with a sense of fulfillment and pleasure.

Constructing a Journey In the same way that an artist builds a masterpiece, we design for ourselves a path of resiliency via the experiences that we have. Combining knowledge, optimistic thinking, self-care, and support from others is the best way to construct a life that is successful in spite of having Ehlers-Danlos syndrome.

In the compelling story that is Ehlers-Danlos Syndrome, each and every one of us plays the role of the main protagonist. As we go forward, we will use knowledge as our compass, self-care as our loving companion, and a support network as our safety net. When we collaborate with people who are already established in the field, we can ensure that we have access to the resources that will be the most helpful to us on our trip. By cultivating mindfulness, developing our advocacy skills, and placing a focus on enjoyment, we increase our ability to adapt and thrive in the world.

Remember that Ehlers-Danlos Syndrome is only one piece of the puzzle, and not the full story by itself; this is important for us to keep in mind. Those of us who have Ehlers-Danlos syndrome navigate the ups and downs of life's journey with tenacity and optimism, seeing each passing second as an opportunity to create a masterpiece that demonstrates our resiliency and vitality. We see each passing second as a chance to create a masterpiece that shows our resilience and vitality.

Printed in Great Britain
by Amazon